YOUR KNOWLEDGE HAS VALUE

- We will publish your bachelor's and master's thesis, essays and papers

- Your own eBook and book - sold worldwide in all relevant shops

- Earn money with each sale

Upload your text at www.GRIN.com and publish for free

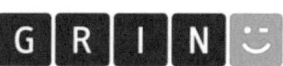

Bibliographic information published by the German National Library:

The German National Library lists this publication in the National Bibliography; detailed bibliographic data are available on the Internet at http://dnb.dnb.de .

This book is copyright material and must not be copied, reproduced, transferred, distributed, leased, licensed or publicly performed or used in any way except as specifically permitted in writing by the publishers, as allowed under the terms and conditions under which it was purchased or as strictly permitted by applicable copyright law. Any unauthorized distribution or use of this text may be a direct infringement of the author s and publisher s rights and those responsible may be liable in law accordingly.

Imprint:

Copyright © 2018 GRIN Verlag
Print and binding: Books on Demand GmbH, Norderstedt Germany
ISBN: 9783668747494

This book at GRIN:

https://www.grin.com/document/432523

Patrick Kimuyu

The Impact of Industrial Farming on the Environment

GRIN Verlag

GRIN - Your knowledge has value

Since its foundation in 1998, GRIN has specialized in publishing academic texts by students, college teachers and other academics as e-book and printed book. The website www.grin.com is an ideal platform for presenting term papers, final papers, scientific essays, dissertations and specialist books.

Visit us on the internet:

http://www.grin.com/

http://www.facebook.com/grincom

http://www.twitter.com/grin_com

Table of Contents

Introduction 2

Impact of Industrial Farming on the Environment 2

Environmental pollution by fertilizers 3

Environmental Contamination by Genetically Modified Seeds 4

Unhealthy Population 4

Ecological Imbalance 6

Climate Change 7

Conclusion 7

References 9

Introduction

Agricultural production has over the years transformed from subsistence farming to more intensive commercial farming. It is apparent that industrial agriculture has been epitomized as an important way of promoting farming efficiency, as well as increasing agricultural production. This has led to increased food sustainability in developed countries. It has also played a significant role in addressing food shortages in developing countries. Although industrial farming has helped to feed more people around the world, it has brought harm to both people and the planet as a whole. Thankfully, biotechnology has begun to make industrial farming more environmentally friendly, and as a nation we need to more fully embrace the revolution it is bringing to agriculture. It is apparent that industrial farming has immense consequences on the environment ranging from environmental pollution to the phenomenon of climate change. Therefore, this paper will provide an aesthetic analysis of the harmful impact of industrial farming on the environment.

Impact of Industrial Farming on the Environment

Industrial farming involves all aspects of feeding, breeding, raising, and processing animals and crop products for the consumption by humans (Winson, 2014). This is a complex subject that involves individuals, private enterprises, large and small corporate consumers, the community, the state and federal regulators, and the general public. Its systems involve the consumption of fossil fuels, topsoil, and water at very unsustainable rates. It has been found to contribute to several forms of environmental degradation, including air and water pollution, depletion of soils, fish die-offs, and diminishing biodiversity. For instance, the production of meat significantly contributes to these problems (Winson, 2014). Producing grains for animals' consumption instead of the direct consumption by humans involves loss of energy and destruction of resources.

It is also argued that the proliferation of the industry-style livestock production has created environmental, as well as public health concerns, including pollution from the large animal wastes and extensive use of antibiotics (Winson, 2014). The extensive use antibiotics make animal fat to contain higher levels of antibiotics and other chemicals that are believed to contribute to the severity of diseases in humans.

Environmental pollution by fertilizers

Foremost, the use of inorganic fertilizers for crop production has been found to increase food production. According to Altieri (1998), an ecological expert, the amounts of nitrogen applied to the most arable lands fluctuate between 120-550 kilograms of nitrogen per hectare. However, the bountiful harvests that are realized as a result of fertilizer application have also been associated with devastating environmental consequences. According to Winson (2014), the increased application of fertilizers leads to high incidences of pests and diseases. It is apparent that crops grown under fertilizer have been found to be susceptible to pests because they have higher foliage levels. As such, they serve as pest harbors for pests that destroy foliage; thus increasing environmental degradation.

Moreover, the wasteful and inappropriate application and utilization of fertilizers by crops lead to environmental pollution. Significant amounts of fertilizers that are not used by crops are normally washed into the surfaces water and groundwater. It is estimated that about 25 percent of groundwater sources such as wells, in America contain high level of nitrate (Winson, 2014). This is attributed to the intensive use of fertilizers in crop production. The high nitrate levels in water are dangerous to human health. According to Heagle et al. (1973), nitrates lower oxygen levels in the children's bloodstream and causes gastric, esophageal, and bladder cancers in adults.

Fertilizers have also been found to destroy aquatic habitats. For instance, excessive use of fertilizers has led to the growth of algal glooms in water bodies such as lakes. When fertilizer residues are washed into lakes by rainfall, phosphorous and nitrogen in these residues favor a phenomenon referred to as eutrophication. In this case, aquatic plants grow rapidly to cause overcrowding and competition for nutrients and sunlight. It is apparent that eutrophication has devastating consequences. Some of these consequences include degradation of recreational opportunities, tainted drinking water supplies and suffocation of aquatic animals including fish. It is reported that eutrophication related damages cost the US about $2.2 billion each year (Chislock, Doster, Zitomer & Wilson, 2013).

Environmental Contamination by Genetically Modified Seeds

Winson (2014) suggests that though some forms of biotechnology have improved crop farming, they still have a potential of being misused if left under the control of multinational corporations. The intrusion of private interest in biotechnology has resulted into devastating environmental and health implications. For instance, there is evidence that some genetically modified seeds are harmful to the environment. Currently, industrial farming has adopted genetically modified crops to increase agricultural production. Therefore, it has facilitated the harmful environmental consequences. Genetically modified seeds have been reported to cause devastating harm to the environment. An outstanding example is the destruction of monarch butterflies by pollen from genetically modified corn that was engineered by Monsanto (Friedlander, 1999).

Unhealthy Population

Industrial agriculture has led to several public health concerns such as antimicrobial resistance, impacts on occupational and community health, and transfer of zoonotic diseases to humans (Marshall & Levy, 2011). Zoonotic diseases are those diseases that are transmitted from animals to humans. It has also been found to cause significant disruptions to ecological balances. Of particular concerns are the industrial farming concentration and its juxtaposition with the general human population. The environmental impacts of industrial farming can be assessed in light of its potential impacts on individuals and the general population. The effects of industrial farming include diseases and disease transmission, with an increased potential for pathogens spreading from the animals to humans.

In some incidences, cases of mental and social health have also been recorded. Many animals are confined in farm structures, which increased the likelihood of animal diseases being easily transmitted to humans as a result of the accumulation of wastes. Animal waste often contains several pathogens when left untreated or when minimally treated. These wastes are usually swept into water bodies when they are applied as fertilizers on farms with poor land management practices. For example, in 2006, animal waste runoff was suspected to have caused *Escherichia coli* outbreak that killed three people and left two hundred sick (Winson, 2014).

Industrial farming has also led to increased food-borne infections. According to Winson (2014), farm produce has a high likelihood of microbial contamination. It has been found to increase microbial contamination of food. Marshall and Levy (2011) explain that meat, dairy, and poultry production, as well as manure handling processes, can lead to food contamination and zoonotic diseases. The occurrence of zoonotic diseases is worsened by industrial farm houses that house livestock. Zoonotic diseases are diseases caused by microbial agents and normally exist in animals, but can be transmitted to human beings (Winson, 2014). According to Gürlük, Uzel, and Turan (2015), of the 1400 documented human pathogens, it is estimated that 64 percent of them are zoonotic. When individuals come into contact with the zoonotic pathogens, they can spread the pathogens to the entire community, thereby leading to adverse effects on the human population.

Moreover, industrial farming also impacts on occupational health. According to Winson (2014), toxic gasses and dust are produced in industrial farm facilities. These substances can cause chronic or temporary respiratory irritation to the farm workers. Many sickness symptoms that grain handlers experience have also been attributed to industrial farming. Such of these health conditions include chronic and acute bronchitis, mucous membrane irritation, non-allergic asthma-like syndrome, and infectious sinusitis. In most cases, these conditions are more severe among smokers than in nonsmokers. It is also worth noting that there is an emerging health condition associated with industrial farming known as Organic Dust Toxic Syndrome (ODTS). This is one of the common infections that are reported among industrial farm workers.

According to Gürlük, Uzel, and Turan (2015), experts in health, industrial agriculture has strong relationships with asthma. In a study carried out by Altieri (2011), it was found out that there was a higher prevalence of asthma, 41%, among children of swine farmers who lived on their farms. It was also found out that there was a higher prevalence of asthma in children who lived on farms that used antibiotics as additives in animal feeds. These results are important because they show that children who live in industrial farms are more vulnerable to asthma as compared to those children who live away from industrialized farms. Therefore, public health professionals and environmentalists in rural areas have the responsibility to pursue environmental measures that seek to eliminate or minimize the risk of asthma among children.

Ecological Imbalance

From an ecological perspective, it is apparent that industrial farming has led to immense ecological imbalance in the ecosystem. Foremost, destruction of wetlands during farming activities has led to loss of habitat for aquatic animal and plant species. Ordinarily, wetlands serve as ecological sites within which organisms that are suited to that environment interact. These interactions enhance energy flow in the ecosystem. Therefore, destruction of wetlands has led to an unprecedented disruption of energy flow in the ecosystem. This implies that some animal and plant species are likely to get extinct.

On the other hand, industrial farming has led to massive contamination of aquatic habitats. For instance, agrochemicals used for spraying crops are usually washed into the water systems. Lakes, rivers and other water bodies around areas where large farms exist experience high levels of contamination with agrochemicals. These chemicals are toxic to aquatic animals such as fish and crustaceans. There have been incidences of fish deaths in rivers that flow through arable land. Moreover, contamination of water sources with agrochemicals causes harm to humans. This is so because people are likely to be poisoned through drinking contaminated water or consumption of food from aquatic sources such as fish.

Climate Change

Bristow and Fitzgerald (2011) observe that industrial farming has been heavily linked to climate change. Industrial farming involves consumption of energy, which result into emission of greenhouse gasses that cause global warming. Winson (2014) explains that industrial livestock farming contributes to 37% of methane, 9% of carbon dioxide, and 65% of nitrous emissions. The industrialized livestock production immensely contributes to anthropogenic carbon (IV) oxide. These emissions directly lead to the destruction of the ozone layer. Furthermore, there is increased pressure on land as a result of increasing population and agricultural activities (Matei-Gherman, 2014). Forests and wetlands are increasingly being cleared to give way for crop and livestock production. These activities have led to the changing rainfall and drought patterns across the world.

Conclusion

In a brief conclusion, it is apparent that industrial farming has devastating consequences to the environment. Foremost, it causes air, water and soil pollution. The fact that industrial farming is highly mechanized implies that machines emit exhaust fumes into the environment; thus causing air pollution. These gases have been reported to cause respiratory health problems. In addition, exhaust fumes contain high levels of greenhouse gases. Therefore, emission of exhaust fumes into the atmosphere has contributed to climate change including global warming and depletion carbon sink zones. On the other hand, excessive use of fertilizers in industrial farming contributes to contamination of water bodies.

Moreover, industrial farming has contributed to antibiotic resistance due to the excessive use of antibiotics on farm animals which are consumed by humans. It has also led to the destruction of the ecosystem through disrupting energy flow, especially in wetlands. This aspect has been found to cause negative consequences to biodiversity including extinction of aquatic species.

Finally, the adoption of biotechnology in industrial farming, especially genetic modification has been found to cause environmental consequences. Some genetically modified seeds cause contamination to the environment as it was witnessed with the modified corn that killed monarch butterflies in the United States. Therefore, industrial farming should be viewed as a double-edged sword; it has immense environmental harm as it shows benefits in food production.

References

Altieri, M. (2011). Modern agriculture: ecological impacts and the possibilities for truly sustainable farming. *Agroecology in Action*. Retrieved from: http://www.mcc.cmu.ac.th/graduate/Agro723/Reading_Materials/Modern_Agri.html

Altieri, M. A. (1998). Ecological impacts of industrial agriculture and the possibilities for truly sustainable farming. *Monthly Review, 50*(3), 60-71.

Bristow, E., & Fitzgerald, A. J. (2011). Global climate change and the industrial animal agriculture link: the construction of risk. *Society & Animals, 19*(3), 205-224.

Chislock, M. F., Doster, E., Zitomer, R. A., & Wilson, A. E. (2013). Eutrophication: Causes, Consequences, and Controls in Aquatic Ecosystems. *Nature Education Knowledge, 4*(4), 10. Retrieved from http://www.nature.com/scitable/knowledge/library/eutrophication-causes-consequences-and-controls-in-aquatic-102364466

Friedlander, B. (1999, April 19). Toxic pollen from widely planted, genetically modified corn can kill monarch butterflies, Cornell study shows. *Cornell Chronicle*. Retrieved from http://www.news.cornell.edu/stories/1999/04/toxic-pollen-bt-corn-can-kill-monarch-butterflies

Gürlük, S., Uzel, G., & Turan, Ö. (2015). Impacts of cattle and sheep husbandry on global greenhouse gas emissions: a time series analysis for central European countries. *Polish Journal of Environmental Studies, 24*(1), 93-98.

Heagle, A. S., Body, D. E., & Heck, W. W. (1973). An open-top field chamber to assess the impact of air pollution on plants. *Journal of Environmental Quality, 2*(3), 365-368

Marshall, B. M., & Levy, S. B. (2011). Food animals and antimicrobials: impacts on human health. *Clinical microbiology reviews, 24*(4), 718-733.

Matei-Gherman, C. (2014). The agriculture ecological need or an experienced. *Agronomy Series of Scientific Research, 57*(1), 219-225.

Notarnicola, B., Hayashi, K., Curran, M. A., & Huisingh, D. (2012). Progress in working towards a more sustainable agri-food industry. *Journal of Cleaner Production, 28*(1), 1-8.

Winson, A. (2014). *The industrial diet: The degradation of food and the struggle for healthy eating*. New York, NY: New York Press.

YOUR KNOWLEDGE HAS VALUE

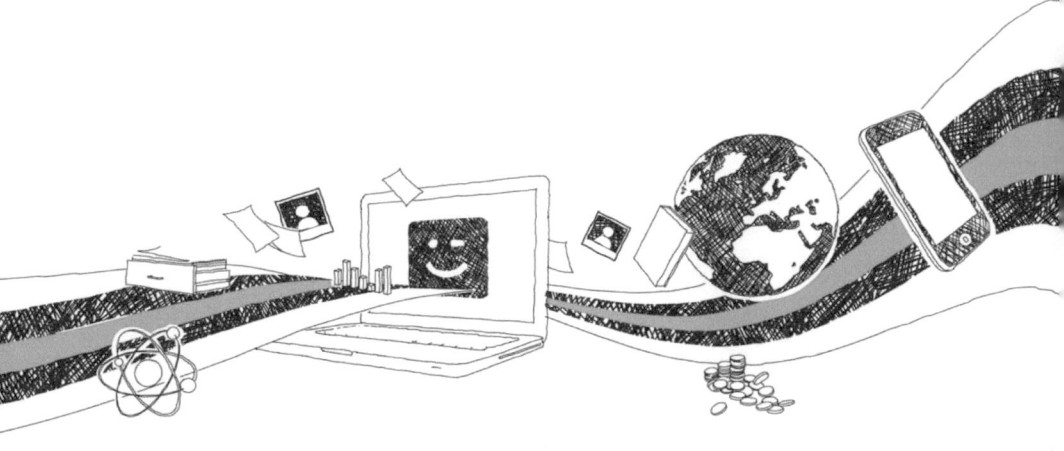

- We will publish your bachelor's and master's thesis, essays and papers

- Your own eBook and book - sold worldwide in all relevant shops

- Earn money with each sale

Upload your text at www.GRIN.com and publish for free

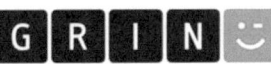